Promoting LGBTQ+ Health and Wellness: A Guide for Healthcare Workers

Copyright Page

TITLE: Promoting LGBTQ+ Health and Wellness: A Guide for Healthcare Workers

1ST Edition

ISBN: 9798223304494

Table of Contents

Promoting LGBTQ+ Health and Wellness: A Guide for Healthcare Workers

By Roberto Miguel Rodriguez

Introduction:

- Briefly introduce the purpose and scope of the book "Promoting LGBTQ+ Health and Wellness: A Guide for Healthcare Workers".

- Highlight the importance of understanding the unique needs and challenges faced by LGBTQ+ individuals in healthcare settings.

- Emphasize that the outline provided is flexible and can be tailored to meet the specific needs and preferences of healthcare workers.

LGBTQ+ History

- Explore the historical context and narratives of homosexuality throughout different cultures and time periods.

- Discuss the impact of historical events on the LGBTQ+ community and healthcare practices.

- Highlight the importance of understanding LGBTQ+ history in providing culturally competent care.

LGBTQ+ Parenting

- Focus on the experiences and challenges faced by homosexual individuals and couples in becoming parents and raising children.

- Discuss the legal and social considerations related to LGBTQ+ parenting.

- Provide guidance and resources for healthcare workers to support LGBTQ+ parents and their children.

LGBTQ+ Mental Health

- Examine the unique mental health concerns and support systems for homosexual individuals.

- Address issues such as coming out, self-acceptance, and discrimination.

- Provide strategies for healthcare workers to promote LGBTQ+ mental health and well-being.

LGBTQ+ Representation in Media

- Analyze the portrayal and representation of homosexual individuals in various forms of media.

- Explore the impact of media on perceptions and attitudes towards LGBTQ+ individuals.

- Discuss the role of healthcare workers in challenging stereotypes and promoting positive representation.

LGBTQ+ Advocacy and Activism

- Discuss the efforts and initiatives taken by homosexual individuals and allies to fight for equal rights, social acceptance, and inclusivity.

- Highlight the role of healthcare workers in supporting LGBTQ+ advocacy and activism.

- Provide resources for healthcare workers to engage in LGBTQ+ advocacy efforts.

LGBTQ+ Intersectionality

- Explore the experiences and challenges faced by individuals who identify as both homosexual and belong to other marginalized communities.

- Discuss the intersection of LGBTQ+ identities with race, religion, disability, and other factors.

- Provide guidance for healthcare workers on providing inclusive and intersectional care.

LGBTQ+ Health and Wellness

- Focus on the specific health concerns, medical needs, and access to healthcare for homosexual individuals.

- Discuss common health disparities and barriers to care faced by LGBTQ+ individuals.

- Provide recommendations for healthcare workers to promote LGBTQ+ health and wellness.

LGBTQ+ Relationships and Dating

- Discuss various aspects of romantic relationships, dating, and intimacy within the homosexual community.

- Address unique challenges and considerations for LGBTQ+ relationships.

- Provide guidance on supporting LGBTQ+ individuals in navigating healthy relationships.

LGBTQ+ Spirituality

- Explore the intersection of homosexuality and various religious or spiritual practices.

- Discuss the experiences and challenges faced by homosexual individuals within different faith communities.

- Provide resources for healthcare workers to support LGBTQ+ individuals in their spiritual journey.

LGBTQ+ Rights and Legislation

- Examine the legal landscape and progress made in terms of LGBTQ+ rights and protections.

- Discuss global and national perspectives on LGBTQ+ rights.

- Highlight the role of healthcare workers in advocating for LGBTQ+ rights and supporting legislative changes.

Conclusion:

- Summarize the key themes and topics covered in the book.

- Reinforce the importance of understanding and addressing the specific needs of LGBTQ+ individuals in healthcare settings.

- Encourage healthcare workers to continuously educate themselves and stay updated on LGBTQ+ health and wellness.

Chapter 1: LGBTQ+ History

Exploring the historical context of homosexuality

Understanding the historical context of homosexuality is essential for healthcare workers in providing culturally competent care to LGBTQ+ individuals. Throughout different cultures and time periods, the experiences and narratives of homosexuality have varied greatly, often shaped by societal norms, religious beliefs, and political landscapes. This subchapter aims to shed light on the historical background of homosexuality, enabling healthcare workers to better comprehend the unique challenges faced by LGBTQ+ individuals.

The chapter begins by delving into LGBTQ+ history, examining how homosexuality has been perceived and understood in different cultures. From ancient civilizations like Greece and Rome, where same-sex relationships were celebrated, to the Middle Ages, when homosexuality was condemned as sinful and criminalized, these historical perspectives have had a profound impact on societal attitudes towards homosexuality.

Furthermore, the subchapter explores LGBTQ+ parenting and the experiences of homosexual individuals and couples in becoming parents and raising children. It delves into the challenges they face, including legal and societal barriers, and highlights the importance of inclusive healthcare practices in supporting LGBTQ+ families.

In discussing LGBTQ+ mental health, the chapter addresses the unique concerns faced by homosexual individuals. It examines the psychological impact of coming out, self-acceptance, and discrimination, and emphasizes the need for healthcare professionals to provide safe spaces and support systems for LGBTQ+ individuals.

The subchapter also delves into LGBTQ+ representation in media, analyzing the portrayal of homosexual individuals across various forms of media. It highlights the importance of accurate and diverse representation in promoting inclusivity and combating stereotypes.

Advocacy and activism within the LGBTQ+ community are also explored, focusing on the efforts made by homosexual individuals and allies to fight for equal rights and social acceptance. The chapter discusses the role of healthcare workers in supporting these initiatives and promoting inclusivity within healthcare settings.

Furthermore, the subchapter explores the intersectionality of LGBTQ+ identities, discussing the experiences and challenges faced by individuals who identify as both homosexual and belong to other marginalized communities. Understanding the unique needs of LGBTQ+ individuals who face multiple forms of discrimination is crucial for providing comprehensive care.

The chapter concludes by examining the specific health concerns and medical needs of homosexual individuals, emphasizing the importance of equal access to healthcare and addressing healthcare disparities within the LGBTQ+ community.

By exploring the historical context of homosexuality, healthcare workers can gain a deeper understanding of LGBTQ+ individuals' experiences, challenges, and needs. This knowledge is crucial in fostering a safe and inclusive healthcare environment that promotes the health and wellness of all individuals, regardless of their sexual orientation.

Homosexuality in ancient civilizations

In this subchapter, we delve into the historical context and narratives surrounding homosexuality in ancient civilizations. Understanding the experiences and treatment of homosexual individuals throughout history is crucial for healthcare workers in providing culturally sensitive and inclusive care to LGBTQ+ patients.

Ancient civilizations, such as ancient Greece, Rome, Egypt, and Mesopotamia, offer valuable insights into the acceptance, tolerance, and even celebration of homosexuality. In ancient Greece, for example, homosexual relationships were common and socially accepted, particularly between adult men and adolescent boys. These relationships were considered a mentorship and a way to pass down knowledge and wisdom.

Similarly, in ancient Rome, same-sex relationships were prevalent, with the term "homosexuality" itself being coined from the Latin word "homos" meaning "same." Emperors like Hadrian and Nero were known for their same-sex relationships, challenging traditional gender norms.

Ancient Egyptian civilization also demonstrated a more fluid understanding of sexuality, with evidence of same-sex relationships depicted in artwork and literature. The pharaohs themselves were often depicted engaging in same-sex relationships, emphasizing the acceptance of homosexuality within their society.

Mesopotamia, known as the cradle of civilization, also had a nuanced approach to homosexuality. The Epic of Gilgamesh, one of the oldest surviving literary works, portrays a deep emotional bond between Gilgamesh and Enkidu, which some scholars interpret as a same-sex relationship.

Exploring the acceptance of homosexuality in ancient civilizations not only challenges the assumption that homosexuality is a modern construct but also highlights the importance of cultural relativism in healthcare. Understanding the historical context of homosexuality can help healthcare workers approach LGBTQ+ patients with empathy and respect, acknowledging the diversity of human experiences throughout time.

By examining these ancient civilizations, healthcare workers can gain insights into the historical acceptance of homosexuality, which can inform their interactions with LGBTQ+ patients today. This knowledge can contribute to creating inclusive healthcare environments that prioritize the mental and physical well-being of all patients, regardless of their sexual orientation or gender identity.

The impact of colonialism and religion on LGBTQ+ history

In order to fully understand the historical context and narratives of homosexuality, it is crucial to examine the impact of colonialism and religion on LGBTQ+ history. This subchapter explores how these two factors have shaped the experiences, struggles, and achievements of the LGBTQ+ community throughout different cultures and time periods.

Colonialism played a significant role in shaping the perception and treatment of homosexuality in many regions around the world. As European powers expanded their empires, they imposed their own cultural norms and values on indigenous communities, often condemning and criminalizing homosexuality. This resulted in the erasure of indigenous LGBTQ+ histories and the imposition of Western heteronormative ideals. The effects of colonialism can still be felt today, as many former colonies continue to grapple with the legacy of these oppressive laws and attitudes.

Religion has also played a significant role in shaping LGBTQ+ history. Many major world religions have historically viewed homosexuality as sinful or immoral, leading to widespread discrimination and persecution of LGBTQ+ individuals. Religious teachings and doctrines have often been used to justify discrimination, violence, and exclusion. However, it is important to note that there are also religious traditions and communities that have embraced and supported LGBTQ+ individuals, challenging the dominant narratives and fostering spaces of acceptance and inclusion.

Understanding the impact of colonialism and religion on LGBTQ+ history is crucial for healthcare workers, as it helps inform their practice and approach to providing healthcare to LGBTQ+ individuals. Many LGBTQ+ individuals face unique challenges when seeking healthcare, including stigma, discrimination, and a lack of culturally competent care. By understanding the historical context and narratives of homosexuality, healthcare workers can better understand these challenges and provide more inclusive and affirming care.

Moreover, healthcare workers have a responsibility to challenge and dismantle the systems of oppression that have contributed to the marginalization of LGBTQ+ individuals. This includes advocating for policy changes, promoting LGBTQ+ rights and protections, and working towards a healthcare system that is inclusive, equitable, and affirming for all individuals, regardless of their sexual orientation or gender identity.

By exploring the impact of colonialism and religion on LGBTQ+ history, healthcare workers can gain a deeper understanding of the unique needs and experiences of LGBTQ+ individuals. This knowledge can inform their practice, improve healthcare outcomes, and contribute to the overall health and wellness of LGBTQ+ individuals and communities.

LGBTQ+ rights movements throughout history

Subchapter: LGBTQ+ Rights Movements Throughout History

Introduction:

LGBTQ+ rights movements have played a crucial role in advocating for equality, social acceptance, and inclusivity for homosexual individuals. This subchapter explores the historical context of these movements, highlighting key milestones and influential figures who have paved the way for progress. By understanding the struggles and achievements of the

LGBTQ+ community, healthcare workers can provide more empathetic and informed care to their patients.

Key Milestones:

The LGBTQ+ rights movements have evolved over time, witnessing significant milestones that have shaped the current landscape. From the Stonewall Riots of 1969, which marked a turning point in the fight for LGBTQ+ rights, to the decriminalization of homosexuality in various countries, such as the United Kingdom in 1967 and Canada in 1969, these events have propelled the movement forward. Additionally, the removal of homosexuality from the Diagnostic and Statistical Manual of Mental Disorders (DSM) in 1973 was a pivotal moment in affirming the legitimacy of homosexuality.

Influential Figures:

Numerous individuals have made significant contributions to LGBTQ+ rights movements throughout history. Figures like Harvey Milk, the first openly gay elected official in California, and Marsha P. Johnson, a transgender activist and key participant in the Stonewall Riots, have become icons of the movement. Their courage and advocacy have paved the way for greater visibility and acceptance.

Global Progress:

The fight for LGBTQ+ rights extends beyond national borders. While progress has been made in some regions, such as the legalization of same-sex marriage in countries like Canada, the United States, and several European nations, challenges persist in other parts of the world. Healthcare workers must be aware of the diverse legal landscapes and cultural contexts that impact the health and well-being of LGBTQ+ individuals globally.

Health Implications:

LGBTQ+ rights movements have gone hand in hand with improvements in LGBTQ+ health and wellness. These movements have helped reduce stigma, increase access to healthcare, and promote culturally competent care for homosexual individuals. However, healthcare workers must remain vigilant in addressing the unique health concerns faced by the LGBTQ+ community, such as higher rates of mental health issues, substance abuse, and sexually transmitted infections.

Conclusion:

Understanding the historical context and achievements of LGBTQ+ rights movements is essential for healthcare workers. By appreciating the struggles and progress of the LGBTQ+ community, healthcare professionals can foster a more inclusive and supportive environment for their patients. Through continued advocacy and awareness, the healthcare system can better meet the specific health needs of LGBTQ+ individuals, promoting their overall well-being and quality of life.

Chapter 2: LGBTQ+ Parenting

Challenges faced by homosexual individuals and couples in becoming parents

Becoming a parent is a deeply personal and rewarding experience, but for homosexual individuals and couples, this journey often comes with unique challenges. In this subchapter, we will explore the experiences and obstacles faced by homosexual individuals and couples in their pursuit of parenthood, shedding light on the healthcare workers' role in supporting them.

One of the primary challenges faced by homosexual individuals and couples is the lack of legal recognition and protection for their parental rights. In many countries, same-sex couples may face legal barriers when it comes to adoption, surrogacy, or accessing assisted reproductive technologies. Healthcare workers, therefore, play a crucial role in advocating for these individuals and couples, ensuring they have access to the necessary resources and support.

Another challenge is the societal stigma and discrimination that homosexual individuals and couples experience when it comes to raising children. They may face judgment from healthcare providers, family members, or even their own children's schools. Healthcare workers must be aware of these biases and strive to create a safe and inclusive environment for all families, regardless of sexual orientation.

Moreover, the financial burden of pursuing parenthood can be significant for homosexual individuals and couples. Adoption, surrogacy, and fertility treatments can be costly, and many insurance policies do not cover these expenses for same-sex couples. Healthcare workers can assist by providing information on financial assistance programs, insurance options, and affordable healthcare resources.

Mental health concerns are also prevalent among homosexual individuals and couples navigating the path to parenthood. The stress of facing discrimination, societal pressure, and the fear of judgment can take a toll on their well-being. Healthcare workers should be equipped to provide mental health support, including counseling services and referrals to LGBTQ+ affirming therapists.

In conclusion, becoming a parent as a homosexual individual or couple presents a unique set of challenges. From legal obstacles to societal stigma, the journey to parenthood requires healthcare workers to be knowledgeable, empathetic, and supportive. By recognizing and addressing these challenges, healthcare workers can play a vital role in promoting the health and well-being of LGBTQ+ individuals and families.

Adoption and foster care for LGBTQ+ individuals

In recent years, there has been a significant shift in societal attitudes towards LGBTQ+ individuals and their rights. One area where this change is particularly evident is in the realm of adoption and foster care. LGBTQ+ individuals and couples are increasingly seeking to become parents and provide loving homes for children in need. However, they continue to face unique challenges and barriers in the adoption and foster care process.

This subchapter aims to provide healthcare workers with a comprehensive understanding of the issues surrounding adoption and foster care for LGBTQ+ individuals. It explores the historical context and narratives of homosexuality, highlighting the progress made in recent years and the ongoing struggles faced by LGBTQ+ individuals in their journey to parenthood.

The chapter delves into the experiences and challenges faced by homosexual individuals and couples in becoming parents and raising children. It examines the legal landscape and progress made in terms of LGBTQ+ rights and protections, both globally and within specific countries. It also addresses the discrimination and prejudice that LGBTQ+ parents may encounter within the adoption and foster care system and provides guidance on how healthcare workers can support them.

Additionally, the subchapter explores the unique mental health concerns of LGBTQ+ individuals seeking to adopt or foster children. It addresses issues such as coming out, self-acceptance, and the impact of discrimination on their well-being. It provides healthcare workers with tools and resources to support the mental health and overall well-being of LGBTQ+ individuals navigating the adoption and foster care process.

Furthermore, the chapter highlights the importance of LGBTQ+ representation in media and its impact on the adoption and foster care system. It discusses the portrayal and representation of homosexual individuals in various forms of media, including film, television, literature, and music, and how these representations can influence societal attitudes towards LGBTQ+ parents.

Ultimately, this subchapter aims to empower healthcare workers to be advocates for LGBTQ+ individuals and couples seeking to become parents through adoption or foster care. It equips them with the knowledge and understanding of the unique challenges faced by LGBTQ+ individuals in the adoption and foster care system, and provides them with the tools and resources to provide inclusive and affirming care.

Assisted reproductive technologies and surrogacy

Assisted reproductive technologies (ART) and surrogacy have become vital options for many LGBTQ+ individuals and couples who wish to become parents. These innovative medical interventions have provided hope and a path to parenthood for those who may not have been able to conceive or carry a child on their own.

ART refers to a range of medical procedures that assist with the conception of a child. These include in vitro fertilization (IVF), intrauterine insemination (IUI), and sperm or egg donation. These methods have allowed same-sex couples to have biological children and experience the joys of parenthood.

Surrogacy, on the other hand, involves a woman carrying a child for another individual or couple. This process can be achieved through traditional surrogacy, where the surrogate's own eggs are used, or gestational surrogacy, where the surrogate carries an embryo created through IVF using the intended parents' or donors' genetic material.

For healthcare workers, it is crucial to be knowledgeable about the unique considerations and challenges faced by LGBTQ+ individuals and couples when it comes to assisted reproductive technologies and surrogacy. Providing inclusive and affirming care requires understanding the specific needs and desires of LGBTQ+ individuals who are seeking to build their families.

Healthcare workers should be aware of the legal and ethical aspects surrounding ART and surrogacy, as they vary by country and jurisdiction. It is important to be familiar with local laws and regulations, as well as any potential obstacles or limitations LGBTQ+ individuals may encounter during their journey towards parenthood.

Additionally, healthcare workers should be sensitive to the emotional and psychological aspects of the assisted reproductive process. The path to parenthood can be complex and emotionally charged for LGBTQ+ individuals and couples. Understanding the unique mental health concerns and support systems for homosexual individuals is crucial in providing comprehensive care.

Furthermore, healthcare workers should be knowledgeable about the potential health concerns and medical needs specific to LGBTQ+ individuals who are using assisted reproductive technologies or engaging in surrogacy. This includes addressing the increased risk of certain health conditions and providing appropriate medical guidance and support throughout the process.

By being well-informed and supportive, healthcare workers can play a vital role in ensuring the health and well-being of LGBTQ+ individuals and couples who are navigating the assisted reproductive journey. Their expertise and understanding can make a significant difference in helping LGBTQ+ individuals achieve their dreams of parenthood while receiving compassionate and affirming care.

Navigating legal and societal barriers in LGBTQ+ parenting

In recent years, there has been significant progress in recognizing and supporting LGBTQ+ families. However, many legal and societal barriers still exist, creating unique challenges for homosexual individuals and couples who want to become parents or raise children. As healthcare workers, it is crucial to understand these barriers and provide appropriate support and resources to LGBTQ+ parents.

One of the primary legal barriers faced by LGBTQ+ parents is adoption and foster care restrictions. While many countries and states have legalized same-sex adoption, others still have discriminatory laws that make it difficult for homosexual individuals and couples to adopt or foster children. This not only denies LGBTQ+ individuals the opportunity to become parents but also denies children the chance to find loving and supportive homes.

Another legal barrier is the lack of recognition for LGBTQ+ families. Many countries do not legally recognize same-sex marriages or partnerships, which can lead to challenges in terms of parental rights, custody, and inheritance. These legal limitations can have a significant impact on the well-being and stability of LGBTQ+ families.

Societal barriers also play a role in the challenges faced by LGBTQ+ parents. Homophobia and discrimination can result in prejudice and stigma, leading to social isolation and limited support networks. LGBTQ+ parents may face judgment and criticism from family members, friends, and even healthcare providers, which can negatively impact their mental health and well-being.

As healthcare workers, it is essential to be aware of these barriers and provide LGBTQ+ parents with the support and resources they need. This includes creating a safe and inclusive environment where they feel comfortable discussing their parenting journey and accessing appropriate healthcare services.

Advocacy and education are key in addressing these barriers. Healthcare workers can engage in LGBTQ+ advocacy efforts, supporting initiatives that aim to change discriminatory laws and promote equality for LGBTQ+ families. Additionally, healthcare providers can educate themselves and their colleagues on LGBTQ+ parenting issues, ensuring that they are knowledgeable and sensitive to the unique needs and challenges faced by LGBTQ+ parents.

By navigating these legal and societal barriers, healthcare workers can play a vital role in supporting LGBTQ+ parents and ensuring their health and well-being, as well as the health and well-being of their children.

Chapter 3: LGBTQ+ Mental Health

Coming out and self-acceptance in the LGBTQ+ community

Coming out and self-acceptance are pivotal moments in the lives of LGBTQ+ individuals, and healthcare workers play a crucial role in supporting their journey towards self-discovery and embracing their identity. This subchapter will delve into the experiences and challenges faced by LGBTQ+ individuals during the coming out process and the importance of self-acceptance for their overall health and well-being.

The coming out process can be a transformative and emotional journey for LGBTQ+ individuals. It involves disclosing their sexual orientation or gender identity to family, friends, and colleagues. Healthcare workers need to understand the significance of this process and be prepared to offer support and guidance to patients who are navigating this path.

Coming out can have a profound impact on an individual's mental health. LGBTQ+ individuals often face fear, anxiety, and the risk of rejection or discrimination when opening up about their identity. Healthcare workers need to be aware of the unique mental health concerns faced by this community, including higher rates of depression, anxiety, and suicidal ideation. By fostering a safe and accepting environment, healthcare professionals can alleviate some of the burdens associated with coming out.

Self-acceptance is an ongoing process that LGBTQ+ individuals must navigate. It involves embracing their identity, developing a positive self-image, and challenging internalized homophobia or transphobia. Healthcare workers can play a vital role in promoting self-acceptance by providing affirming care and connecting patients with support networks, such as LGBTQ+ community organizations or therapy groups.

Furthermore, healthcare workers need to be knowledgeable about the specific health concerns faced by LGBTQ+ individuals. This includes understanding the increased risk of certain health conditions, such as HIV/AIDS, mental health disorders, and substance abuse, as well as the barriers to accessing healthcare services that this community often encounters. By addressing these unique health needs, healthcare professionals can contribute to the overall well-being of LGBTQ+ individuals.

In conclusion, coming out and self-acceptance are essential aspects of the LGBTQ+ experience. Healthcare workers have a responsibility to create a safe and supportive environment for individuals going through the coming out process and to promote self-acceptance as a foundation for improved mental and physical health. By gaining a deeper understanding of the challenges faced by LGBTQ+ individuals, healthcare workers can contribute to a more inclusive and affirming healthcare system for all.

Discrimination and its impact on mental health

In this subchapter, we will delve into the profound impact of discrimination on the mental health of LGBTQ+ individuals. As healthcare workers, it is crucial for us to understand the unique challenges faced by this community in order to provide effective support and care.

Discrimination against LGBTQ+ individuals is still prevalent in many societies, leading to significant mental health disparities. When individuals face rejection, prejudice, and harassment based on their sexual orientation or gender identity, it can result in increased levels of anxiety, depression, and even suicide. The constant fear of being judged or mistreated can create a hostile environment that takes a toll on one's psychological well-being.

One of the key contributors to mental health struggles within the LGBTQ+ community is the process of coming out. While it can be liberating for some, for others, it brings immense stress and fear of rejection from loved ones or society at large. Healthcare workers need to be sensitive and provide a safe space for individuals navigating this journey, offering resources and support to help them cope with the potential mental health challenges.

Moreover, LGBTQ+ individuals often face discrimination within healthcare systems themselves. This can lead to avoidance of seeking medical care, resulting in delayed or inadequate treatment for physical and mental health issues. As healthcare workers, it is our responsibility to create an inclusive and welcoming environment, free from bias and judgment, to ensure LGBTQ+ individuals receive the care they deserve.

Addressing discrimination and its impact on mental health requires a multidimensional approach. Healthcare workers can play a vital role in advocating for LGBTQ+ rights and challenging discriminatory practices. By staying up-to-date with the legal landscape and legislation surrounding LGBTQ+ rights, we can actively support initiatives that promote equal rights, social acceptance, and inclusivity for all individuals.

In conclusion, discrimination against LGBTQ+ individuals has a profound impact on their mental health. By understanding and addressing the unique challenges faced by this community, healthcare workers can provide the support and care needed to promote their mental well-being. It is our duty to advocate for equal rights, challenge discriminatory practices, and create inclusive healthcare environments that prioritize the mental health and overall well-being of LGBTQ+ individuals.

LGBTQ+ support systems and resources

LGBTQ+ support systems and resources play a crucial role in promoting the health and wellness of individuals within the LGBTQ+ community. Healthcare workers have a responsibility to be aware of these support systems and resources in order to provide comprehensive and inclusive care to their LGBTQ+ patients.

Understanding the historical context and narratives of homosexuality is essential for healthcare workers when working with LGBTQ+ patients. Exploring the rich history of LGBTQ+ individuals throughout different cultures and time periods can provide valuable insights into the challenges they have faced and the progress that has been made.

In the context of LGBTQ+ parenting, healthcare workers should be knowledgeable about the experiences and challenges faced by homosexual individuals and couples in becoming parents and raising children. This includes awareness of adoption and surrogacy options, legal considerations, and support networks available to LGBTQ+ parents.

LGBTQ+ mental health is a critical aspect of overall well-being. Healthcare workers need to be familiar with the unique mental health concerns of homosexual individuals, including issues such as coming out, self-acceptance, and discrimination. Understanding the support systems available, such as LGBTQ+ counseling services and support groups, can help healthcare workers provide appropriate care and referrals.

Representation in media has a powerful impact on societal attitudes towards homosexuality. Healthcare workers should critically analyze the portrayal and representation of homosexual individuals in various forms of media, including film, television, literature, and music. This understanding can help challenge stereotypes and promote positive representation.

Advocacy and activism are vital components of the LGBTQ+ movement. Healthcare workers should be aware of the efforts and initiatives taken by homosexual individuals and allies to fight for equal rights, social acceptance, and inclusivity. This knowledge can help healthcare workers support their LGBTQ+ patients and contribute to a more inclusive healthcare system.

LGBTQ+ intersectionality recognizes that individuals may belong to multiple marginalized communities. Healthcare workers should explore the experiences and challenges faced by individuals who identify as both homosexual and belong to other marginalized communities, such as race, religion, or disability. This understanding can help healthcare workers provide culturally competent and inclusive care.

LGBTQ+ health and wellness encompass the specific health concerns, medical needs, and access to healthcare for homosexual individuals. Healthcare workers should be knowledgeable about LGBTQ+ health disparities, including higher rates of mental health issues, substance abuse, and sexually transmitted infections. They should also be aware of LGBTQ+ healthcare providers and LGBTQ+ friendly healthcare facilities.

Understanding the dynamics of LGBTQ+ relationships and dating is important for healthcare workers. They should have knowledge about various aspects of romantic relationships, dating, and intimacy within the homosexual community. This understanding can help healthcare workers provide appropriate sexual health education and support.

LGBTQ+ spirituality is a complex and diverse topic. Healthcare workers should explore the intersection of homosexuality and various religious or spiritual practices and be sensitive to the experiences and challenges faced by homosexual individuals within different faith communities. This understanding can help healthcare workers provide holistic care that respects spiritual beliefs.

Finally, healthcare workers should be aware of LGBTQ+ rights and legislation. They should examine the legal landscape and progress made in terms of LGBTQ+ rights and protections, both globally and within specific countries. This knowledge can help healthcare workers advocate for their LGBTQ+ patients and ensure they receive equal and respectful treatment.

By being well-informed about LGBTQ+ support systems and resources, healthcare workers can provide compassionate and inclusive care to their LGBTQ+ patients.

Mental health concerns specific to LGBTQ+ individuals

Introduction:

In this subchapter, we will delve into the unique mental health concerns faced by LGBTQ+ individuals. As healthcare workers, it is crucial to understand and provide appropriate support for this population. LGBTQ+ individuals often experience higher rates of mental health issues due to societal stigma, discrimination, and the challenges associated with coming out and self-acceptance.

The Impact of Stigma and Discrimination:

Stigma and discrimination can have a profound impact on the mental well-being of LGBTQ+ individuals. Rejection from family and friends, bullying, and societal prejudice contribute to higher rates of anxiety, depression, and suicidal ideation. Healthcare workers must create a safe and inclusive environment to address these concerns.

Coming Out and Self-Acceptance:

Coming out is a significant milestone for many LGBTQ+ individuals. It is a process that involves self-discovery, acceptance, and potential challenges. Healthcare workers should be prepared to provide support during this journey, offering resources and counseling services to navigate the emotional and psychological aspects of coming out.

Addressing Internalized Homophobia:

Internalized homophobia refers to the self-hatred or negative feelings that LGBTQ+ individuals may internalize due to societal stigma. These feelings can lead to low self-esteem, anxiety, and depression. Healthcare workers can play a vital role in helping individuals challenge and overcome internalized homophobia through therapy and support.

Discrimination in Healthcare:

LGBTQ+ individuals often face discrimination within healthcare settings, making it challenging for them to seek appropriate care. Healthcare workers must be aware of the specific needs of LGBTQ+ patients and provide culturally competent care. This includes using inclusive language, understanding the unique health risks faced by this population, and being knowledgeable about LGBTQ+ resources and support networks.

Intersectionality and Mental Health:

LGBTQ+ individuals who also belong to other marginalized communities may face compounded challenges. Healthcare workers should be aware of the intersectionality of identities and the impact it can have on mental health. Understanding the experiences of LGBTQ+ individuals who are also racial or religious minorities, disabled, or of different socioeconomic backgrounds is crucial for providing effective care.

Conclusion:

Mental health concerns specific to LGBTQ+ individuals are complex and require healthcare workers to be sensitive, knowledgeable, and supportive. By understanding the impact of stigma, discrimination, and the challenges associated with self-acceptance, healthcare professionals can play a crucial role in promoting the mental well-being of LGBTQ+ individuals. Through inclusive and culturally competent care, we can help create a society where LGBTQ+ individuals can thrive mentally, emotionally, and physically.

Chapter 4: LGBTQ+ Representation in Media

Portrayal of homosexuality in film

In recent years, there has been a significant shift in the portrayal of homosexuality in film, challenging stereotypes and providing a more nuanced representation of LGBTQ+ individuals. This subchapter will explore the evolution of this portrayal and its impact on healthcare workers' understanding of LGBTQ+ health and wellness.

Historically, homosexuality in film was often depicted negatively, reinforcing harmful stereotypes and perpetuating discrimination. LGBTQ+ characters were often portrayed as deviant, tragic, or objects of ridicule, contributing to the stigmatization and marginalization of the community. However, with the rise of LGBTQ+ activism and advocacy, filmmakers have increasingly embraced more authentic and positive portrayals of homosexuality.

Today, LGBTQ+ characters are being represented in a variety of genres, allowing for a more diverse and accurate reflection of the community. This includes films that explore LGBTQ+ history, such as "Milk," which tells the story of Harvey Milk, one of the first openly gay elected officials in the United States. By highlighting the struggles and triumphs of historical figures, these films provide healthcare workers with a deeper understanding of the challenges faced by LGBTQ+ individuals throughout history.

Moreover, films centered around LGBTQ+ parenting, like "The Kids Are All Right," provide healthcare workers with valuable insights into the unique experiences and challenges faced by homosexual individuals and couples in becoming parents and raising children. These films shed light on issues such as adoption, surrogacy, and co-parenting, allowing healthcare workers to better support LGBTQ+ parents.

In terms of mental health, the portrayal of homosexuality in film has a significant impact on self-acceptance and coming out experiences. Films like "Moonlight" and "Love, Simon" depict the struggles faced by LGBTQ+ individuals in accepting their sexual orientation and coming out to their friends and family. By showcasing these experiences, healthcare workers can better understand the mental health concerns specific to the LGBTQ+ community, as well as the importance of providing support and resources for self-acceptance.

Furthermore, the representation of LGBTQ+ individuals in film contributes to the broader movement for LGBTQ+ rights and social acceptance. Films like "Brokeback Mountain" and "Carol" portray LGBTQ+ relationships with depth and sensitivity, challenging societal norms and promoting empathy and understanding. Healthcare workers can learn from these films about the dynamics of LGBTQ+ relationships and the importance of inclusivity and acceptance in promoting the health and wellness of LGBTQ+ individuals.

In conclusion, the portrayal of homosexuality in film has undergone significant changes over the years, moving away from harmful stereotypes and providing more authentic and positive representations. By exploring these films, healthcare workers can gain a better understanding of LGBTQ+ history, parenting challenges, mental health concerns, and relationship dynamics within the community. This knowledge is crucial in providing inclusive and affirming care to LGBTQ+ individuals, promoting their health and wellness.

LGBTQ+ characters in television shows and series

LGBTQ+ representation in television shows and series has played a significant role in shaping societal attitudes and perceptions towards the community. From groundbreaking characters to nuanced storylines, these portrayals have contributed to increased visibility, acceptance, and understanding of LGBTQ+ individuals. As healthcare workers, it is crucial to recognize and appreciate the impact of LGBTQ+ representation in media and its implications for the health and well-being of our patients.

Television shows and series have increasingly included LGBTQ+ characters, allowing viewers to see diverse and authentic representations of sexual orientation and gender identity. These characters often navigate various life experiences, including coming out, forming relationships, and dealing with discrimination. By showcasing the challenges and triumphs of LGBTQ+ individuals, television programs have the power to educate and humanize their stories, fostering empathy and understanding among viewers.

For healthcare workers, understanding LGBTQ+ representation in television shows and series is essential for providing culturally competent care. By engaging with media that features LGBTQ+ characters, healthcare workers can gain insights into the unique health concerns, mental health issues, and support systems that are specific to this community. It allows us to empathize with the experiences of our patients, creating a safe and inclusive space for them to seek healthcare services.

Moreover, LGBTQ+ representation in television shows and series can also inspire and empower individuals within the community. Seeing characters who resemble their own experiences can help LGBTQ+ individuals feel seen, validated, and less alone. This, in turn, can positively impact mental health outcomes, self-acceptance, and overall well-being.

However, it is important to critically analyze LGBTQ+ representation in media to ensure that it avoids harmful stereotypes or tokenism. While progress has been made in recent years, there is still work to be done to ensure that LGBTQ+ characters are authentically portrayed and given substantial storylines beyond their sexual orientation or gender identity.

In conclusion, LGBTQ+ characters in television shows and series have contributed to increased visibility, acceptance, and understanding of the community. As healthcare workers, engaging with LGBTQ+ representation in media can enhance our cultural competency and understanding of the unique health concerns faced by LGBTQ+ individuals. By recognizing the power of media in shaping attitudes and perceptions, we can create a more inclusive and supportive healthcare environment for all patients.

Representation in literature and poetry

Representation in literature and poetry plays a crucial role in promoting LGBTQ+ health and wellness. By exploring diverse narratives and experiences, healthcare workers can gain a deeper understanding of the challenges faced by homosexual individuals and develop more inclusive and informed approaches to care.

Literature and poetry have long been powerful tools for reflecting and shaping societal attitudes towards homosexuality. From ancient texts to contemporary works, these forms of expression have provided LGBTQ+ individuals with a means of self-discovery, self-acceptance, and validation. However, representation has not always been positive or accurate, and healthcare workers need to be aware of the historical context and biases that may be present in the literature they encounter.

By delving into LGBTQ+ literature and poetry, healthcare workers can gain insights into the historical context and narratives of homosexuality throughout different cultures and time periods. This understanding allows them to provide culturally competent care and recognize the unique challenges faced by LGBTQ+ individuals in different societal contexts.

Furthermore, literature and poetry can shed light on the experiences and challenges faced by homosexual individuals and couples in becoming parents and raising children. By exploring LGBTQ+ parenting narratives, healthcare workers can better support these individuals and address their specific needs, such as family planning, fertility treatments, and navigating legal and societal barriers.

Representation in literature and poetry also provides a platform for discussing mental health concerns within the LGBTQ+ community. Works that explore topics such as coming out, self-acceptance, and discrimination can help healthcare workers understand the unique stressors faced by homosexual individuals and develop appropriate interventions and support systems.

Moreover, analyzing the portrayal and representation of homosexual individuals in various forms of media, including literature, film, television, and music, allows healthcare workers to critically examine societal attitudes and stereotypes that may impact the health and well-being of LGBTQ+ individuals. By understanding the influence of media on perceptions and self-image, healthcare workers can challenge harmful narratives and promote positive representation.

In conclusion, representation in literature and poetry is a valuable tool for healthcare workers in promoting LGBTQ+ health and wellness. By exploring historical narratives, parenting experiences, mental health concerns, media representation, and more, healthcare workers can develop a more comprehensive and inclusive approach to care for LGBTQ+ individuals.

LGBTQ+ musicians and their impact on society

In recent years, LGBTQ+ musicians have played a significant role in shaping and influencing society. Through their music and public persona, these artists have challenged societal norms, advocated for LGBTQ+ rights, and provided a voice for marginalized communities. This subchapter will explore the impact of LGBTQ+ musicians on society, highlighting their contributions to LGBTQ+ history, mental health, representation in media, advocacy and activism, and the intersections of their identities with other marginalized communities.

Throughout history, LGBTQ+ musicians have been instrumental in shaping the cultural landscape. From iconic figures like Freddie Mercury and Elton John to contemporary artists like Sam Smith and Janelle Monáe, their music has resonated with diverse audiences, breaking barriers and challenging stereotypes. By openly embracing their sexuality and sharing their personal journeys, these musicians have become role models for the LGBTQ+ community, inspiring self-acceptance and promoting mental health.

Representation in media is crucial for fostering understanding and acceptance, and LGBTQ+ musicians have been at the forefront of this movement. Their visibility in music videos, interviews, and performances has helped normalize homosexuality, challenging prejudices and promoting inclusivity. By showcasing diverse relationships and experiences through their lyrics, LGBTQ+ musicians have given voice to the community's struggles, joys, and triumphs.

Beyond their music, LGBTQ+ musicians have also been powerful advocates and activists. They have used their platforms to speak out against discrimination, support LGBTQ+ rights, and raise awareness about important issues. From participating in Pride events to organizing benefit concerts, these musicians have played a pivotal role in advancing the fight for equal rights and social acceptance.

The intersectionality of LGBTQ+ identities is another important aspect to consider. LGBTQ+ musicians who belong to other marginalized communities, such as racial, religious, or disabled communities, face unique challenges. They navigate multiple identities, often facing discrimination and experiencing complex forms of oppression. Understanding these intersections is crucial for healthcare workers to provide culturally competent care and support.

In conclusion, LGBTQ+ musicians have had a profound impact on society, shaping LGBTQ+ history, challenging societal norms, and amplifying the voices of marginalized communities. Their contributions to mental health, representation in media, advocacy and activism, and intersectionality cannot be overstated. As healthcare workers, it is essential to recognize and understand the influence of LGBTQ+ musicians in order to provide comprehensive and inclusive care to LGBTQ+ individuals.

Chapter 5: LGBTQ+ Advocacy and Activism

Historical milestones in LGBTQ+ advocacy

Throughout history, LGBTQ+ individuals and their allies have worked tirelessly to advocate for equal rights, social acceptance, and inclusivity. These efforts have paved the way for significant advancements in LGBTQ+ rights and have shaped the landscape of healthcare, mental health, parenting, representation in media, and more. This subchapter will explore some of the key historical milestones in LGBTQ+ advocacy that healthcare workers should be aware of.

One of the earliest milestones in LGBTQ+ advocacy can be traced back to the mid-19th century when the first organized homosexual rights organizations emerged in Europe. The Scientific-Humanitarian Committee, founded in Berlin in 1897, was one such organization that sought to decriminalize homosexuality and promote tolerance.

The Stonewall Riots of 1969 in New York City marked a turning point in LGBTQ+ advocacy. Following a police raid on the Stonewall Inn, a popular gay bar, the LGBTQ+ community fought back against the discriminatory treatment they faced. This event sparked a wave of activism and led to the formation of numerous LGBTQ+ organizations and pride parades around the world.

In the 1970s, LGBTQ+ activists began demanding recognition and protection under the law. The American Psychiatric Association, for example, removed homosexuality from its list of mental disorders in 1973, challenging harmful stereotypes and contributing to the advancement of LGBTQ+ mental health.

The 1980s and 1990s were marked by the devastating AIDS epidemic, which disproportionately affected the LGBTQ+ community. This crisis sparked a wave of activism, with organizations such as ACT UP (AIDS Coalition to Unleash Power) advocating for increased research, access to healthcare, and an end to discrimination.

In the early 2000s, the fight for marriage equality gained momentum. In 2001, the Netherlands became the first country to legalize same-sex marriage, and this milestone was followed by numerous others around the world. The legalization of same-sex marriage not only granted LGBTQ+ individuals the right to marry but also had significant implications for healthcare, parenting, and legal recognition.

Recent years have seen increased visibility and awareness of LGBTQ+ issues, thanks in part to the power of social media and the efforts of LGBTQ+ activists. The legalization of same-sex marriage in the United States in 2015 and the repeal of the "Don't Ask, Don't Tell" policy in the military are just a few examples of the progress made in LGBTQ+ rights and legislation.

Understanding these historical milestones is essential for healthcare workers to provide culturally competent and inclusive care to LGBTQ+ individuals. By acknowledging the struggles, triumphs, and ongoing challenges faced by the LGBTQ+ community, healthcare workers can play a vital role in promoting LGBTQ+ health and wellness.

Allyship and support for LGBTQ+ rights

In recent years, there has been a growing recognition of the rights and needs of the LGBTQ+ community. As healthcare workers, it is crucial for us to actively support and advocate for the rights of our LGBTQ+ patients. This subchapter explores allyship and support for LGBTQ+ rights, providing healthcare workers with the knowledge and tools to create a safe and inclusive environment for all individuals.

Allyship is the practice of individuals from privileged groups actively supporting and advocating for marginalized communities. For healthcare workers, allyship entails recognizing the unique challenges faced by LGBTQ+ individuals and taking steps to address and mitigate them. This includes creating a welcoming and affirming environment, using inclusive language, and educating oneself on LGBTQ+ health issues.

Supporting LGBTQ+ rights also involves understanding the historical context and narratives of homosexuality throughout different cultures and time periods. By exploring LGBTQ+ history, healthcare workers can gain valuable insights into the struggles and achievements of the community, fostering empathy and understanding.

Furthermore, this subchapter delves into the experiences and challenges faced by LGBTQ+ individuals in various aspects of their lives. From LGBTQ+ parenting to mental health concerns, representation in media, and intersectionality, healthcare workers will gain a comprehensive understanding of the unique needs and experiences of LGBTQ+ individuals. This knowledge will enable them to provide culturally competent and sensitive care, ensuring that LGBTQ+ patients feel understood and supported.

Additionally, healthcare workers will learn about LGBTQ+ advocacy and activism, examining the efforts made by the community and its allies to fight for equal rights, social acceptance, and inclusivity. By understanding these initiatives, healthcare workers can become allies themselves, actively participating in the movement for LGBTQ+ rights.

Finally, this subchapter explores the legal landscape surrounding LGBTQ+ rights and protections. By examining global and country-specific legislation, healthcare workers can advocate for policy changes that promote equality and non-discrimination in healthcare settings.

In conclusion, allyship and support for LGBTQ+ rights is a fundamental aspect of providing inclusive and equitable healthcare. By educating ourselves on LGBTQ+ history, understanding the unique challenges faced by the community, and actively advocating for their rights, healthcare workers can foster a safe and welcoming environment for all patients.

Intersectionality in LGBTQ+ activism

Intersectionality in LGBTQ+ activism is a crucial concept that healthcare workers need to understand in order to provide inclusive and effective care for all patients. It acknowledges that individuals can face multiple forms of oppression and discrimination based on their various intersecting identities, such as race, religion, disability, or socioeconomic status, in addition to their sexual orientation or gender identity.

In LGBTQ+ activism, intersectionality recognizes that the experiences and challenges faced by homosexual individuals can be further compounded by their other marginalized identities. For example, a person who is both gay and a person of color may face racism within the LGBTQ+ community or experience homophobia within their racial or ethnic community. This intersectional perspective emphasizes the need to address and dismantle all forms of discrimination and inequality.

By understanding intersectionality, healthcare workers can better support LGBTQ+ individuals in their unique struggles. For instance, they can provide culturally competent care by recognizing how discrimination may impact the mental health of LGBTQ+ individuals, particularly those who belong to multiple marginalized communities. Healthcare providers can also advocate for policies and practices that promote inclusivity, such as ensuring equal access to healthcare services, regardless of a person's intersecting identities.

Additionally, intersectionality prompts healthcare workers to critically examine their own biases and privilege. They can challenge assumptions and stereotypes, and actively seek to create a safe and affirming environment for LGBTQ+ individuals from all walks of life. By acknowledging and addressing the intersecting oppressions faced by LGBTQ+ individuals, healthcare workers can contribute to a more just and equitable society.

In summary, intersectionality is a crucial lens through which to approach LGBTQ+ activism. By recognizing and addressing the unique challenges faced by individuals who identify as both homosexual and belong to other marginalized communities, healthcare workers can provide more inclusive and effective care. Understanding intersectionality is essential for creating a healthcare system that meets the diverse needs of LGBTQ+ individuals and promotes their health and well-being.

Current initiatives and future directions in advocacy

Advocacy plays a crucial role in advancing the rights and well-being of the LGBTQ+ community. Over the years, there have been numerous initiatives and movements that have shaped the landscape of LGBTQ+ advocacy. This subchapter explores the current initiatives and future directions in advocacy that are aimed at promoting LGBTQ+ health and wellness. By addressing the specific concerns and challenges faced by the LGBTQ+ community, healthcare workers can play a vital role in creating a more inclusive and affirming healthcare environment.

One significant initiative in LGBTQ+ advocacy is the push for comprehensive LGBTQ+ healthcare training for healthcare professionals. Recognizing the unique health needs and disparities faced by LGBTQ+ individuals, organizations and institutions are increasingly offering educational programs and resources to healthcare workers. These initiatives focus on increasing awareness and understanding of

LGBTQ+ health issues, including mental health concerns, access to healthcare, and cultural competency.

Another important direction in advocacy is the promotion of LGBTQ+ inclusive policies and practices within healthcare settings. This includes advocating for policies that protect against discrimination based on sexual orientation and gender identity, as well as policies that ensure LGBTQ+ individuals have access to appropriate and affirming healthcare services. Healthcare workers can play a crucial role in advocating for these policies within their own institutions and collaborating with LGBTQ+ advocacy organizations to promote change at a broader level.

Furthermore, there is a growing emphasis on intersectionality within LGBTQ+ advocacy. Recognizing that LGBTQ+ individuals often face multiple forms of marginalization, such as racism, ableism, or religious discrimination, advocacy efforts are increasingly focusing on addressing these intersecting identities. This includes advocating for the inclusion of LGBTQ+ individuals in broader social justice movements and working towards more inclusive policies and legislation that take into account the unique experiences of LGBTQ+ individuals with intersecting identities.

Looking towards the future, there is a need for continued advocacy to address ongoing challenges faced by the LGBTQ+ community. This includes advocating for improved access to gender-affirming healthcare, mental health support, and comprehensive sexual education that is inclusive of LGBTQ+ experiences. Additionally, there is a need for ongoing advocacy to address the disparities faced by LGBTQ+ individuals in healthcare outcomes, such as higher rates of substance abuse, suicide, and HIV/AIDS.

In conclusion, current initiatives and future directions in LGBTQ+ advocacy aim to promote the health and wellness of the LGBTQ+ community. By advocating for comprehensive healthcare training, inclusive policies, intersectionality, and addressing ongoing challenges, healthcare workers can contribute to creating a more inclusive and affirming healthcare environment for LGBTQ+ individuals.

Chapter 6: LGBTQ+ Intersectionality

Experiences of LGBTQ+ individuals belonging to marginalized communities

In this subchapter, we will delve into the experiences of LGBTQ+ individuals who also belong to marginalized communities. These individuals face unique challenges and intersecting forms of discrimination based on their sexual orientation as well as other aspects of their identity, such as race, religion, or disability. As healthcare workers, it is essential to understand and address these challenges in order to provide inclusive and effective care.

Intersectionality plays a significant role in the lives of LGBTQ+ individuals from marginalized communities. They often experience compounded discrimination, facing not only homophobia and transphobia but also racism, religious intolerance, ableism, and other forms of oppression. These intersecting identities shape their experiences of coming out, self-acceptance, and navigating healthcare systems.

For instance, LGBTQ+ individuals who belong to racial or ethnic minority communities may face cultural barriers when seeking healthcare services. They may encounter prejudice or lack of understanding from healthcare providers who are not culturally competent. Moreover, the fear of discrimination and stigmatization may deter them from seeking essential healthcare, resulting in health disparities within this population.

In addition, LGBTQ+ individuals with disabilities may encounter barriers in accessing appropriate care due to physical or communication barriers. Healthcare facilities and providers must prioritize accessibility and provide inclusive care that addresses the unique needs of these individuals.

Addressing the experiences of LGBTQ+ individuals from marginalized communities requires a multifaceted approach. Healthcare workers must educate themselves on the specific challenges faced by these individuals and work towards creating safe and inclusive environments. This includes fostering cultural competence, providing LGBTQ+-affirming care, and advocating for policies that protect the rights and well-being of all patients, regardless of their sexual orientation or other marginalized identities.

Collaboration with community organizations and LGBTQ+ advocacy groups is crucial in understanding the nuances of these experiences and developing tailored interventions. By actively engaging with these communities and listening to their voices, healthcare workers can ensure that their care practices are inclusive and responsive to the needs of LGBTQ+ individuals from marginalized communities.

In conclusion, the experiences of LGBTQ+ individuals from marginalized communities are shaped by intersecting forms of discrimination and oppression. As healthcare workers, it is vital to acknowledge and address these challenges in order to provide equitable and effective care. By fostering cultural competence, advocating for LGBTQ+ rights, and collaborating with community organizations, healthcare workers can contribute to the well-being and resilience of LGBTQ+ individuals from marginalized communities.

The intersection of race and sexuality

The intersection of race and sexuality is a complex and multifaceted topic that requires careful examination and understanding. In this subchapter, we will explore the unique experiences and challenges faced by individuals who identify as both homosexual and belong to racial or ethnic minority groups. This intersectionality is crucial to consider when providing healthcare services to LGBTQ+ individuals, as it significantly impacts their health and wellness.

Historically, racial and ethnic minority communities have faced systemic discrimination and marginalization, and this discrimination often extends to LGBTQ+ individuals within these communities. Healthcare workers need to be aware of the specific health concerns faced by LGBTQ+ individuals of color and the barriers they may encounter when seeking care. For example, transgender people of color have higher rates of HIV infection and face increased levels of violence and discrimination.

Understanding the historical context and narratives of homosexuality within different cultures and time periods is essential in providing culturally sensitive care. By recognizing and respecting the cultural values and beliefs of LGBTQ+ individuals from diverse racial backgrounds, healthcare workers can create a safe and inclusive environment for them.

Furthermore, healthcare workers need to be aware of the unique mental health concerns faced by LGBTQ+ individuals of color. These concerns may include higher rates of depression, anxiety, and suicide due to the experience of multiple forms of discrimination and prejudice. By providing appropriate mental health support, healthcare workers can help LGBTQ+ individuals of color navigate these challenges and promote their overall well-being.

Additionally, it is crucial to address the representation of LGBTQ+ individuals of color in media and ensure their stories are accurately portrayed and heard. By analyzing the portrayal and representation of LGBTQ+ individuals of color in various forms of media, healthcare workers can challenge stereotypes and promote diversity and inclusivity.

Overall, the intersection of race and sexuality plays a significant role in the health and well-being of LGBTQ+ individuals. By understanding and addressing the unique experiences and challenges faced by individuals who identify as both homosexual and belong to racial or ethnic minority groups, healthcare workers can provide more effective and culturally competent care.

LGBTQ+ individuals with disabilities

Subchapter: LGBTQ+ Individuals with Disabilities

Introduction:

In this subchapter, we will explore the unique experiences and challenges faced by LGBTQ+ individuals with disabilities. We will discuss the intersectionality of these identities and how it impacts their health, relationships, mental well-being, and access to healthcare. As healthcare workers, it is crucial to understand and address the specific needs of this diverse group, ensuring inclusivity and equal care for all.

Understanding Intersectionality:

LGBTQ+ individuals with disabilities face compounded challenges due to the intersection of their sexual orientation or gender identity and their disability. This intersectionality often leads to increased discrimination, marginalization, and limited access to resources and support.

Health Concerns and Medical Needs:

LGBTQ+ individuals with disabilities may have unique health concerns and medical needs. Healthcare workers must be aware of these issues, including the higher risk of mental health disorders, chronic conditions, and barriers to healthcare services. Providing inclusive and accessible care is essential to promote their overall health and well-being.

Navigating Relationships and Intimacy:

LGBTQ+ individuals with disabilities may encounter additional barriers when navigating relationships and intimacy. Healthcare workers should be knowledgeable about the challenges they face in forming and maintaining romantic relationships, exploring sexuality, and accessing appropriate sexual health resources.

Access to Healthcare:

Discrimination and ableism can create significant barriers for LGBTQ+ individuals with disabilities when accessing healthcare services. Healthcare workers must actively work towards providing accessible facilities, inclusive policies, and culturally competent care to ensure equitable access to healthcare for all.

Advocacy and Support:

Healthcare workers play a vital role in advocating for the rights and needs of LGBTQ+ individuals with disabilities. By actively supporting initiatives that promote inclusivity, equal rights, and social acceptance, healthcare professionals can contribute to creating a more inclusive society.

Conclusion:

Understanding the unique experiences of LGBTQ+ individuals with disabilities is crucial for healthcare workers. By recognizing the intersectionality of these identities and addressing specific health concerns, access to healthcare, and barriers to relationships and intimacy, healthcare workers can provide more inclusive and equitable care for this marginalized group. Let us strive to create healthcare systems that honor diversity, promote inclusivity, and ensure the well-being of all individuals, regardless of their sexual orientation, gender identity, or disability status.

Religious and cultural challenges faced by LGBTQ+ individuals

In this subchapter, we will explore the religious and cultural challenges that LGBTQ+ individuals often face in their lives. It is essential for healthcare workers to have an understanding of these challenges in order to provide appropriate care and support to this population.

Throughout history, LGBTQ+ individuals have faced persecution and discrimination based on religious beliefs and cultural norms. Many religions have traditionally condemned homosexuality, categorizing it as sinful or immoral. This has led to a significant struggle for LGBTQ+ individuals who are deeply connected to their faith but also grappling with their sexual orientation or gender identity.

In various cultures, homosexuality has been stigmatized and often viewed as a deviation from societal norms. LGBTQ+ individuals may face rejection, isolation, and even violence within their own families and communities due to cultural expectations and prejudices.

These religious and cultural challenges can have adverse effects on the mental health and well-being of LGBTQ+ individuals. They may experience high levels of stress, anxiety, and depression as they navigate the conflict between their sexual orientation or gender identity and their religious or cultural beliefs. Coming out to their families or religious communities can be particularly challenging, as it often leads to strained relationships and even ostracization.

Healthcare workers play a crucial role in supporting LGBTQ+ individuals facing these challenges. By providing a safe and non-judgmental environment, healthcare professionals can help LGBTQ+ patients feel comfortable discussing their religious and cultural concerns. It is important to approach these conversations with empathy and respect, acknowledging the complexity of their identity and the potential conflicts they may be experiencing.

Healthcare workers can also educate themselves on different religious and cultural perspectives on LGBTQ+ issues. This knowledge can enable them to provide appropriate guidance and support while respecting the patient's spiritual or cultural beliefs. It is essential to be aware of resources and support networks within the community that can assist LGBTQ+ individuals in reconciling their sexual orientation or gender identity with their religious or cultural backgrounds.

By addressing the religious and cultural challenges faced by LGBTQ+ individuals, healthcare workers can contribute to their overall health and well-being. Through understanding, compassion, and culturally sensitive care, healthcare professionals can help LGBTQ+ patients navigate the complexities of their identity while maintaining their faith and cultural connections.

Chapter 7: LGBTQ+ Health and Wellness

Unique health concerns for LGBTQ+ individuals

The health and wellness of LGBTQ+ individuals are influenced by a range of factors that are unique to their experiences and identities. Healthcare workers have a crucial role to play in understanding and addressing these specific health concerns. This subchapter aims to provide healthcare workers with insights into the unique health concerns faced by LGBTQ+ individuals, equipping them with the knowledge and tools to provide inclusive and effective care.

One of the key health concerns for LGBTQ+ individuals is mental health. Due to societal stigma, discrimination, and prejudice, LGBTQ+ individuals may experience higher rates of anxiety, depression, and suicide ideation compared to their heterosexual counterparts. Healthcare workers need to be aware of these disparities and provide a supportive environment for LGBTQ+ individuals to discuss their mental health concerns. This may involve creating safe spaces, using affirming language, and being knowledgeable about LGBTQ+ resources and support systems.

Another important aspect of LGBTQ+ health is sexual health. LGBTQ+ individuals may have unique sexual health needs and risks that healthcare workers need to be familiar with. For example, gay and bisexual men may be at a higher risk for sexually transmitted infections, including HIV. Transgender individuals may require specialized care related to hormone therapy and gender-affirming surgeries. It is essential for healthcare workers to provide comprehensive sexual health education and services that are inclusive and non-judgmental.

Additionally, LGBTQ+ individuals may face barriers to accessing appropriate healthcare. These barriers can include lack of knowledge about LGBTQ+ inclusive healthcare providers, fear of discrimination or mistreatment, and financial constraints. Healthcare workers need to be aware of these barriers and work towards creating a welcoming and inclusive environment for LGBTQ+ patients.

Moreover, healthcare workers should be knowledgeable about the unique health concerns faced by LGBTQ+ youth and older adults. LGBTQ+ youth may experience higher rates of homelessness, substance abuse, and self-harm, while older LGBTQ+ adults may face challenges related to social isolation and healthcare disparities. By understanding these specific concerns, healthcare workers can provide tailored care that addresses the unique needs of these populations.

In conclusion, addressing the unique health concerns of LGBTQ+ individuals is vital for healthcare workers. By understanding the mental health disparities, sexual health needs, barriers to healthcare access, and specific concerns of LGBTQ+ youth and older adults, healthcare workers can provide inclusive and effective care. By promoting LGBTQ+ health and wellness, healthcare workers play an essential role in ensuring that all individuals, regardless of their sexual orientation or gender identity, receive the care they need and deserve.

Access to healthcare and healthcare disparities

In this subchapter, we will explore the topic of access to healthcare and healthcare disparities within the LGBTQ+ community. As healthcare workers, it is crucial to understand the unique challenges faced by homosexual individuals when seeking healthcare services and to work towards creating a more inclusive and equitable healthcare system.

It is well-documented that LGBTQ+ individuals face significant healthcare disparities compared to their heterosexual counterparts. These disparities can be attributed to a variety of factors, including discrimination, stigma, and lack of cultural competence among healthcare providers. As a result, many LGBTQ+ individuals face barriers to accessing appropriate and timely healthcare, leading to poorer health outcomes.

One of the primary challenges faced by homosexual individuals is the fear of discrimination and mistreatment when seeking healthcare services. Studies have shown that LGBTQ+ individuals are more likely to experience verbal harassment, refusal of care, and even physical violence in healthcare settings. This fear often leads to a delay in seeking necessary medical care, which can have serious consequences for their health.

Moreover, healthcare providers may lack the knowledge and cultural competence to address the specific health needs of LGBTQ+ individuals. This includes understanding the unique health concerns, such as higher rates of mental health disorders, substance abuse, and certain types of cancers within the LGBTQ+ community. It also involves creating a safe and affirming environment for patients to disclose their sexual orientation or gender identity without fear of judgment or discrimination.

To address these challenges, healthcare workers must undergo comprehensive training on LGBTQ+ health issues and cultural competence. This includes understanding the specific health needs of homosexual individuals, learning appropriate language and terminology, and cultivating a non-judgmental and inclusive approach to care.

Additionally, healthcare organizations and policymakers must work towards implementing policies and practices that promote LGBTQ+ inclusive healthcare. This includes advocating for non-discrimination laws, implementing inclusive patient intake forms, and ensuring that healthcare facilities have LGBTQ+ competent providers. It is also essential to collaborate with LGBTQ+ community organizations to better understand the needs and concerns of the community.

By addressing these healthcare disparities and improving access to care, healthcare workers can play a vital role in promoting the health and well-being of LGBTQ+ individuals. By creating a safe and inclusive healthcare environment, we can ensure that all individuals, regardless of their sexual orientation or gender identity, have equal access to high-quality healthcare services.

LGBTQ+ inclusive healthcare practices

Chapter 6: LGBTQ+ Inclusive Healthcare Practices

In recent years, there has been a growing recognition of the unique healthcare needs and challenges faced by the LGBTQ+ community. As healthcare workers, it is essential for us to provide inclusive and sensitive care to all individuals, regardless of their sexual orientation or gender identity. This subchapter will explore LGBTQ+ inclusive healthcare practices, highlighting the importance of creating safe and affirming spaces for LGBTQ+ patients.

Understanding LGBTQ+ Health Disparities:

To provide effective care, it is crucial to be aware of the specific health disparities faced by LGBTQ+ individuals. Studies have shown that they have higher rates of mental health issues, substance abuse, and certain chronic conditions. Discrimination and stigma within healthcare settings can also contribute to these disparities. By acknowledging and addressing these disparities, healthcare workers can play a vital role in improving the health outcomes of LGBTQ+ patients.

Creating Inclusive Healthcare Environments:

Creating an inclusive healthcare environment is essential for LGBTQ+ patients to feel comfortable and respected. This includes using inclusive language, displaying LGBTQ+ affirming signage, and training staff on LGBTQ+ cultural competency. Healthcare workers should also be knowledgeable about LGBTQ+ resources and support networks within the community to provide appropriate referrals and resources when needed.

Addressing LGBTQ+ Health Concerns:

LGBTQ+ individuals have unique health concerns that need to be addressed in a sensitive manner. These concerns may include sexual health, hormone replacement therapy, gender-affirming surgeries, and mental health support. Healthcare workers should familiarize themselves with LGBTQ+ health guidelines and best practices to ensure that they are providing appropriate and comprehensive care.

Building Trust and Allies:

As healthcare workers, it is essential to build trust and establish ourselves as allies to the LGBTQ+ community. This can be achieved by actively listening to patients, showing empathy, and advocating for their rights and well-being. By creating a safe and supportive space, healthcare workers can help LGBTQ+ individuals feel more comfortable disclosing their identities and seeking necessary care.

Engaging in LGBTQ+ Advocacy:

Advocacy for LGBTQ+ rights and healthcare is crucial for creating lasting change. Healthcare workers can engage in advocacy efforts by supporting LGBTQ+ organizations, participating in community events, and staying informed about LGBTQ+ legislation and policies. By taking an active role in advocacy, healthcare workers can contribute to the fight for equal rights and access to healthcare for all.

In conclusion, LGBTQ+ inclusive healthcare practices are essential for providing equitable and effective care to all individuals. By understanding the specific health needs and challenges faced by the LGBTQ+ community, healthcare workers can create safe and affirming spaces, address health disparities, and advocate for LGBTQ+ rights. Together, we can work towards a future where every LGBTQ+ individual receives the care and support they deserve.

Mental, sexual, and reproductive healthcare needs

In this subchapter, we will delve into the unique mental, sexual, and reproductive healthcare needs of LGBTQ+ individuals. As healthcare workers, it is crucial for us to understand and address these needs to provide comprehensive and inclusive care.

Mental healthcare is a vital aspect of LGBTQ+ health and wellness. Homosexual individuals often face higher rates of mental health concerns due to societal stigma, discrimination, and the challenges of coming out and self-acceptance. As healthcare providers, it is essential to create a safe and supportive environment for patients to discuss their mental health concerns openly. We will explore strategies to promote mental well-being, including counseling, support groups, and referral services.

Sexual and reproductive healthcare is another crucial component of LGBTQ+ healthcare. Many homosexual individuals encounter unique challenges and barriers when seeking sexual and reproductive services. It is important for healthcare workers to be knowledgeable about LGBTQ+-inclusive sexual health practices, contraception options, and sexually transmitted infection prevention and treatment. We will discuss strategies for providing culturally competent care, including taking a comprehensive sexual history and using inclusive language.

Additionally, this section will address the specific reproductive healthcare needs of LGBTQ+ individuals. Same-sex couples and transgender individuals may require assistance with fertility options, adoption, and assisted reproductive technologies. As healthcare workers, we must be aware of the resources available and provide guidance and support to LGBTQ+ individuals and couples navigating the path to parenthood.

Through this subchapter, healthcare workers will gain a deeper understanding of the mental, sexual, and reproductive healthcare needs of LGBTQ+ individuals. By embracing LGBTQ+ inclusive practices, we can ensure that all patients receive the care they deserve, free from stigma and discrimination.

Chapter 8: LGBTQ+ Relationships and Dating

Building healthy relationships in the LGBTQ+ community

Building healthy relationships in the LGBTQ+ community is a crucial aspect of promoting overall health and wellness for individuals who identify as lesbian, gay, bisexual, transgender, or queer. As healthcare workers, it is essential to understand the unique challenges and experiences faced by LGBTQ+ individuals in their relationships, as well as how to provide support and guidance.

In order to build healthy relationships within the LGBTQ+ community, it is important to create a safe and inclusive environment where individuals feel comfortable expressing their identities and desires. This can be achieved by using inclusive language, avoiding assumptions about gender or sexual orientation, and being knowledgeable about LGBTQ+ history and culture.

Understanding the historical context and narratives of homosexuality throughout different cultures and time periods is crucial in order to challenge societal norms and stereotypes that may negatively impact LGBTQ+ relationships. By familiarizing ourselves with the struggles and victories of past generations, healthcare workers can better support individuals in their journey towards healthy relationships.

LGBTQ+ relationships can face unique challenges, particularly in regards to parenting and raising children. Healthcare workers should be aware of the experiences and challenges faced by homosexual individuals and couples in becoming parents, as well as the specific needs and concerns of LGBTQ+ families. Providing resources and support for LGBTQ+ parents can help them navigate the complexities of family life and create a nurturing environment for their children.

Mental health is also a crucial aspect of building healthy relationships in the LGBTQ+ community. LGBTQ+ individuals often face higher rates of mental health concerns, such as depression, anxiety, and substance abuse. Healthcare workers should be knowledgeable about these issues and provide appropriate support and resources. Additionally, addressing issues such as coming out, self-acceptance, and discrimination are essential in helping LGBTQ+ individuals develop healthy relationships with themselves and others.

Representation in media plays a significant role in shaping societal attitudes towards homosexuality, which in turn impacts LGBTQ+ relationships. Healthcare workers should critically analyze the portrayal and representation of homosexual individuals in various forms of media and be aware of the potential impact on their patients' self-esteem and relationship dynamics.

Advocacy and activism are vital in the fight for equal rights and social acceptance for the LGBTQ+ community. Healthcare workers can support LGBTQ+ individuals by being allies and actively working towards creating inclusive healthcare environments and policies.

Lastly, healthcare workers should recognize the intersectionality of LGBTQ+ identities with other marginalized communities such as race, religion, or disability. Understanding these intersecting identities is essential in providing sensitive and effective healthcare for LGBTQ+ individuals.

In conclusion, building healthy relationships in the LGBTQ+ community requires a deep understanding of the unique challenges and experiences faced by individuals within this community. By being knowledgeable about LGBTQ+ history, parenting, mental health, representation in media, advocacy, intersectionality, and the specific health concerns of LGBTQ+ individuals, healthcare workers can provide the support and guidance needed to foster healthy relationships within this community.

Navigating dating apps and online platforms

In today's digital age, dating apps and online platforms have become a popular way for individuals to meet and connect with potential partners. This is no different for the LGBTQ+ community, who often turn to these platforms to find meaningful relationships. However, healthcare workers need to be aware of the unique challenges and considerations that may arise when it comes to navigating dating apps and online platforms for LGBTQ+ individuals.

First and foremost, it is important for healthcare workers to understand the potential mental health concerns that may accompany the use of dating apps and online platforms. For many LGBTQ+ individuals, these platforms can be a source of validation, connection, and support. However, they can also be a breeding ground for discrimination, harassment, and rejection. Therefore, healthcare workers should be prepared to address issues related to self-acceptance, coming out, and dealing with discrimination that may arise from these platforms.

Moreover, healthcare workers should be knowledgeable about the specific health concerns and medical needs that may be relevant to LGBTQ+ individuals using dating apps and online platforms. For example, they should be prepared to provide information and resources regarding sexual health, HIV/STI prevention, and the importance of regular testing. They should also be equipped to address the unique challenges that may arise for LGBTQ+ individuals navigating relationships and dating, such as negotiating consent, healthy communication, and maintaining emotional well-being.

Additionally, healthcare workers should be aware of the potential risks and safety concerns that may accompany the use of dating apps and online platforms. LGBTQ+ individuals may face a higher risk of experiencing intimate partner violence, stalking, or blackmail due to their sexual orientation or gender identity. Healthcare workers should be able to provide resources and guidance on how to maintain personal safety, recognize warning signs of abusive behavior, and seek support if needed.

Lastly, healthcare workers should be knowledgeable about the importance of LGBTQ+ representation and inclusivity within dating apps and online platforms. They should advocate for platforms that prioritize the safety, well-being, and rights of LGBTQ+ individuals and encourage their patients to use platforms that align with their values and needs.

In conclusion, navigating dating apps and online platforms can be both exciting and challenging for LGBTQ+ individuals. As healthcare workers, it is important to be informed and prepared to address the unique mental health concerns, health needs, and safety considerations that may arise from using these platforms. By providing support, resources, and guidance, healthcare workers can play a vital role in promoting the health and well-being of LGBTQ+ individuals in the world of online dating.

Intimacy and sexual health within LGBTQ+ relationships

In this subchapter, we will delve into the unique aspects of intimacy and sexual health within LGBTQ+ relationships. As healthcare workers, it is essential to understand and address the specific needs and concerns of individuals within the LGBTQ+ community when it comes to their intimate relationships.

Firstly, it is important to recognize that LGBTQ+ relationships are just as diverse as heterosexual relationships. They come in various forms, including same-sex relationships, transgender relationships, and non-binary relationships. Each of these relationships may have their own particular dynamics and challenges.

One crucial aspect of intimacy within LGBTQ+ relationships is the concept of consent and communication. Just like in any relationship, open and honest communication is key. However, LGBTQ+ individuals may face additional barriers in expressing their desires or boundaries due to societal stigma or discomfort. Healthcare workers can play a vital role in creating a safe environment for patients to discuss their sexual health and provide support in navigating these conversations.

Another important consideration is sexual health and well-being. LGBTQ+ individuals may have specific health needs related to sexual practices, such as the prevention of sexually transmitted infections (STIs) or the management of HIV/AIDS. Healthcare workers should be knowledgeable about the unique risks and challenges faced by LGBTQ+ individuals and provide appropriate education, testing, and treatment options.

Additionally, it is crucial to address the mental health aspects of intimate relationships within the LGBTQ+ community. Many individuals may face internalized homophobia, discrimination, or rejection from families or communities, which can impact their self-esteem and overall well-being. Healthcare workers should be prepared to provide support and resources for mental health concerns, including therapy, support groups, or LGBTQ+ affirming resources.

Overall, understanding the nuances of intimacy and sexual health within LGBTQ+ relationships is essential for healthcare workers to provide comprehensive and affirming care. By being knowledgeable, empathetic, and inclusive, healthcare professionals can foster a safe and supportive environment for LGBTQ+ individuals to address their intimate and sexual health needs.

Addressing relationship challenges and seeking support

In this subchapter, we will delve into the unique relationship challenges faced by LGBTQ+ individuals and provide guidance on how healthcare workers can offer support in navigating these issues. LGBTQ+ individuals encounter a range of relationship dynamics, from dating and intimacy to long-term partnerships and parenting. Understanding and addressing these challenges is crucial for healthcare workers to provide effective care and support to this community.

We will explore the experiences and challenges faced by LGBTQ+ individuals in forming and maintaining relationships, including the impact of societal stigma, discrimination, and internalized homophobia. By examining the historical context and narratives of homosexuality throughout different cultures and time periods, healthcare workers can gain a deeper understanding of the complexities faced by LGBTQ+ individuals in their relationships.

We will also discuss the specific challenges faced by LGBTQ+ individuals in parenting and raising children. From the process of becoming parents to navigating the legal and social complexities of LGBTQ+ parenting, healthcare workers can play a vital role in providing resources, support, and guidance to individuals and couples who are starting or raising a family.

Furthermore, we will explore the impact of these relationship challenges on LGBTQ+ mental health. Coming out, self-acceptance, and discrimination can significantly impact the emotional well-being of individuals in LGBTQ+ relationships. Healthcare workers can learn about the unique mental health concerns faced by this community and develop strategies for providing support and resources to promote their overall well-being.

Finally, we will discuss the importance of seeking support and establishing networks within the LGBTQ+ community. Healthcare workers can provide guidance on accessing LGBTQ+ support groups, counseling services, and community centers that can offer a safe and understanding environment for individuals and couples.

By addressing relationship challenges and offering support, healthcare workers can contribute to the overall health and wellness of LGBTQ+ individuals. By understanding the historical context, unique mental health concerns, and specific challenges faced by this community in forming and maintaining relationships, healthcare workers can provide effective and inclusive care to LGBTQ+ individuals and couples.

Chapter 9: LGBTQ+ Spirituality

Understanding the intersection of homosexuality and spirituality

In this subchapter, we will delve into the complex and often misunderstood relationship between homosexuality and spirituality. As healthcare workers, it is crucial to have a comprehensive understanding of the experiences and challenges faced by homosexual individuals within different faith communities.

Throughout history, homosexuality has been viewed differently across various cultures and time periods. Exploring LGBTQ+ history will provide valuable insights into the historical context and narratives surrounding homosexuality. From ancient civilizations that celebrated same-sex relationships to the persecution and discrimination faced by LGBTQ+ individuals in more recent times, understanding the historical journey is essential in providing compassionate and culturally sensitive care.

Homosexual individuals and couples who desire to become parents and raise children often face unique challenges. LGBTQ+ parenting involves navigating legal, social, and emotional hurdles, with healthcare workers playing a vital role in providing support and guidance throughout the process.

The intersection of homosexuality and mental health is an area of concern that demands our attention. Homosexual individuals may face higher rates of depression, anxiety, and substance abuse due to the challenges of coming out, self-acceptance, and discrimination. Healthcare workers must be equipped with the knowledge and resources to address these specific mental health concerns and provide appropriate support systems.

Media representation plays a significant role in shaping societal attitudes towards homosexuality. Analyzing the portrayal of homosexual individuals in film, television, literature, and music allows healthcare workers to critically examine stereotypes and biases, promoting inclusivity and understanding.

Advocacy and activism are integral to the fight for equal rights and social acceptance for the LGBTQ+ community. Understanding the efforts taken by homosexual individuals and allies helps healthcare workers provide informed and empathetic care.

Intersectionality is a crucial concept when discussing homosexuality. Exploring the experiences and challenges faced by individuals who identify as both homosexual and belong to other marginalized communities, such as race, religion, or disability, will enhance our understanding of the unique struggles they may encounter.

Healthcare workers must also be aware of the specific health concerns, medical needs, and access to healthcare for homosexual individuals. By addressing LGBTQ+ health and wellness, we can work towards eliminating healthcare disparities and providing inclusive and affirming care.

Romantic relationships, dating, and intimacy within the homosexual community have their own dynamics and challenges. Understanding these aspects will enable healthcare workers to provide appropriate support and guidance in areas such as sexual health and relationship counseling.

Lastly, we will explore the intersection of homosexuality and spirituality. This section will delve into the experiences and challenges faced by homosexual individuals within different faith communities. It is essential to understand how religious or spiritual practices can impact the well-being and self-acceptance of LGBTQ+ individuals.

By understanding the intersection of homosexuality and spirituality, healthcare workers can provide affirming and inclusive care that respects an individual's religious or spiritual beliefs while addressing their unique health needs.

Experiences of LGBTQ+ individuals within different faith communities

"Experiences of LGBTQ+ individuals within different faith communities"

In this subchapter, we will explore the experiences of LGBTQ+ individuals within different faith communities. Religion and spirituality play a significant role in many people's lives, but for LGBTQ+ individuals, their faith can be a source of both love and acceptance, as well as discrimination and exclusion. As healthcare workers, it is crucial to have an understanding of these experiences to provide inclusive and culturally sensitive care.

Across cultures and time periods, LGBTQ+ individuals have faced varying degrees of acceptance within different faith communities. Some religious traditions have evolved to be more inclusive, embracing and affirming LGBTQ+ individuals as part of their community. Others, however, continue to hold conservative beliefs that view homosexuality as sinful or immoral.

For LGBTQ+ individuals who identify with a particular faith, the impact of their religious beliefs on their mental health and well-being can be profound. Coming out within a religious context can be especially challenging, as individuals may fear rejection, discrimination, or even expulsion from their faith community. This fear can lead to internalized homophobia, self-doubt, and mental health issues.

Furthermore, LGBTQ+ individuals may struggle with reconciling their sexual orientation or gender identity with the teachings of their faith. They may question whether their identity is compatible with their religious beliefs, and this conflict can lead to feelings of guilt, shame, and a loss of spiritual connection.

In this subchapter, we will also explore the efforts and initiatives taken by LGBTQ+ individuals and allies within different faith communities to promote inclusivity and acceptance. We will discuss the importance of LGBTQ+ advocacy and activism within religious contexts, and how these movements have contributed to positive change.

Finally, we will provide healthcare workers with practical strategies for supporting LGBTQ+ individuals within different faith communities. This includes creating safe and affirming healthcare environments, understanding the unique challenges faced by LGBTQ+ individuals of faith, and providing appropriate mental health support and resources.

By gaining a deeper understanding of the experiences of LGBTQ+ individuals within different faith communities, healthcare workers can provide compassionate and culturally competent care that addresses the specific needs and challenges faced by this population.

Challenges and acceptance in religious settings

Religion plays a significant role in the lives of many individuals, providing them with a sense of purpose, community, and spiritual guidance. However, for LGBTQ+ individuals, religious settings can often become sources of challenge and conflict. This subchapter explores the unique experiences and obstacles faced by homosexual individuals within different faith communities, as well as the potential for acceptance and inclusion.

In many religious traditions, homosexuality has historically been stigmatized and condemned. LGBTQ+ individuals may face rejection, discrimination, and even exclusion from their religious communities. This can lead to feelings of isolation, shame, and a conflict between their sexual orientation and their religious beliefs. Healthcare workers need to be aware of these challenges and provide a safe and non-judgmental space for LGBTQ+ individuals to discuss their experiences.

Despite these challenges, there are also stories of acceptance and progress within religious settings. Many religious leaders and communities have started to engage in dialogue and reflection on LGBTQ+ issues, striving to create more inclusive spaces. Healthcare workers can play a vital role in facilitating this dialogue, providing resources and support to religious communities seeking to become more affirming.

Moreover, it is important to recognize that not all religious communities hold negative views towards homosexuality. Some faith traditions embrace LGBTQ+ individuals and actively work towards building inclusive spaces. Healthcare workers should be aware of these affirming communities and connect LGBTQ+ individuals with them, promoting a sense of belonging and acceptance.

Navigating the intersection of homosexuality and spirituality can be a deeply personal journey for LGBTQ+ individuals. Healthcare workers should approach this topic with sensitivity, acknowledging the potential conflicts and challenges that may arise. This subchapter will provide healthcare workers with insights and strategies for supporting LGBTQ+ individuals in their spiritual journeys, including resources for finding affirming religious communities and addressing the internal struggle between sexual orientation and religious beliefs.

By exploring the challenges and acceptance in religious settings, healthcare workers can better understand the unique experiences of LGBTQ+ individuals within different faith communities. This knowledge will enable them to provide more inclusive and affirming care, addressing the specific needs and concerns of LGBTQ+ individuals navigating their spirituality alongside their sexual orientation.

Nurturing LGBTQ+ spirituality and finding a sense of belonging

In a society that often struggles to accept and embrace diverse identities, LGBTQ+ individuals face unique challenges when it comes to spirituality and finding a sense of belonging. Many faith communities have historically been unwelcoming or even hostile towards homosexuality, causing LGBTQ+ individuals to feel alienated and disconnected from their own spiritual journeys. However, there is growing recognition and support for LGBTQ+ individuals within various religious and spiritual traditions, providing a space for nurturing their spirituality and finding a sense of belonging.

Exploring the intersection of homosexuality and various religious or spiritual practices is crucial for healthcare workers to understand the experiences and challenges faced by LGBTQ+ individuals within different faith communities. By promoting LGBTQ+ health and wellness, healthcare workers can play a vital role in helping individuals reconcile their sexual orientation with their spiritual beliefs, ultimately fostering a sense of belonging and well-being.

One important aspect to consider is the historical context and narratives of homosexuality throughout different cultures and time periods. This exploration allows healthcare workers to gain a deeper understanding of the diverse ways in which LGBTQ+ individuals have been viewed and treated within different religious and spiritual traditions. By understanding the historical background, healthcare workers can better support LGBTQ+ individuals in navigating their spiritual journeys.

Moreover, healthcare workers can play a crucial role in advocacy and activism within faith communities. By educating religious leaders about LGBTQ+ health concerns and advocating for inclusive practices, healthcare workers can help create safe spaces for LGBTQ+ individuals to explore and nurture their spirituality. This can involve challenging discriminatory beliefs and practices, promoting dialogue and understanding, and encouraging a more inclusive interpretation of religious texts.

In addition, healthcare workers can provide support for LGBTQ+ individuals who may be struggling with self-acceptance, coming out, and discrimination within their faith communities. By providing LGBTQ+ mental health support, healthcare workers can help individuals navigate the complex emotions and challenges that may arise when reconciling their sexual orientation with their spiritual beliefs.

Ultimately, nurturing LGBTQ+ spirituality and finding a sense of belonging requires a collaborative effort between healthcare workers, faith communities, and LGBTQ+ individuals themselves. By promoting dialogue, education, and inclusivity, healthcare workers can contribute to creating a more accepting and supportive environment for LGBTQ+ individuals within their spiritual journeys, allowing them to thrive both mentally and spiritually.

Chapter 10: LGBTQ+ Rights and Legislation

Global perspectives on LGBTQ+ rights

Understanding the global perspectives on LGBTQ+ rights is crucial for healthcare workers in order to provide inclusive and sensitive care to their LGBTQ+ patients. This subchapter delves into the historical context, legal landscape, and social acceptance of homosexuality across different cultures and time periods.

Through an exploration of LGBTQ+ history, healthcare workers gain a deeper understanding of the struggles and triumphs of the LGBTQ+ community throughout time. By learning about the experiences of LGBTQ+ individuals in different cultures, healthcare workers can better appreciate the diverse challenges faced by their patients. This knowledge allows healthcare workers to provide culturally competent care that respects the unique needs and experiences of LGBTQ+ individuals from various backgrounds.

The subchapter also delves into the progress made in terms of LGBTQ+ rights and protections globally. By examining the legal landscape, healthcare workers can understand the different rights and protections afforded to LGBTQ+ individuals in different countries. This knowledge is crucial for healthcare workers who may encounter LGBTQ+ patients from different parts of the world, as it helps them navigate the legal, social, and cultural factors that impact their patients' lives.

Furthermore, the subchapter addresses the unique mental health concerns faced by LGBTQ+ individuals, including issues such as coming out, self-acceptance, and discrimination. It explores the support systems available to LGBTQ+ individuals and provides guidance for healthcare workers on how to address these mental health concerns in a compassionate and inclusive manner.

In addition, the subchapter touches on LGBTQ+ advocacy and activism, highlighting the efforts and initiatives taken by LGBTQ+ individuals and allies to fight for equal rights, social acceptance, and inclusivity. Healthcare workers can gain insights into the important role they can play in supporting and advocating for their LGBTQ+ patients within the healthcare system.

By exploring LGBTQ+ rights and legislation both globally and within specific countries, healthcare workers can stay informed about the legal protections and challenges faced by LGBTQ+ individuals. This knowledge enables healthcare workers to provide informed and supportive care and to advocate for policies and practices that promote equality and inclusivity within their healthcare settings.

In conclusion, this subchapter provides healthcare workers with a comprehensive understanding of global perspectives on LGBTQ+ rights. By exploring LGBTQ+ history, mental health concerns, representation in media, intersectionality, and other crucial topics, healthcare workers are equipped to provide compassionate and inclusive care to their LGBTQ+ patients. They are also empowered to advocate for LGBTQ+ rights and equal access to healthcare within their professional roles.

Progress and setbacks in LGBTQ+ rights movements

The LGBTQ+ rights movement has witnessed significant progress over the years, along with several setbacks that have shaped the landscape of equality and acceptance for homosexual individuals. This subchapter will explore the historical context of the movement, highlighting key milestones and examining the challenges that still persist today.

The LGBTQ+ rights movement traces its roots back to the late 19th and early 20th centuries when the first organizations advocating for homosexual rights began to emerge. From the Stonewall Riots in 1969, which marked a turning point in the fight for LGBTQ+ rights, to the decriminalization of homosexuality in various countries, including the United States, progress has been made in dismantling discriminatory laws and policies.

However, setbacks continue to hinder the full realization of LGBTQ+ rights. Discrimination, stigma, and violence against the LGBTQ+ community persist worldwide. Many countries still criminalize same-sex relationships, and individuals face persecution and even death for their sexual orientation or gender identity. Additionally, transgender individuals face unique challenges, including limited access to healthcare and high rates of discrimination and violence.

Healthcare workers play a crucial role in supporting the LGBTQ+ community. By understanding the historical struggles and achievements of the LGBTQ+ rights movement, healthcare professionals can provide compassionate and inclusive care. It is essential to recognize the specific health concerns and medical needs of homosexual individuals, such as mental health issues related to coming out, self-acceptance, and discrimination.

Advocacy and activism within the LGBTQ+ community have played a pivotal role in driving progress. By highlighting the efforts and initiatives taken by homosexual individuals and allies, healthcare workers can better understand the social, cultural, and legal barriers that impact LGBTQ+ individuals' health and well-being.

Understanding the intersectionality of LGBTQ+ identities is also crucial. Individuals who identify as both homosexual and belong to other marginalized communities, such as race, religion, or disability, face compounded challenges. Healthcare workers must recognize and address these unique experiences to provide comprehensive care.

While progress has been made in LGBTQ+ rights and legislation, there is still much work to be done. By staying informed about the legal landscape and advocating for equal rights and protections, healthcare workers can contribute to a more inclusive and accepting society.

In conclusion, the LGBTQ+ rights movement has experienced both progress and setbacks throughout history. Healthcare workers have a responsibility to understand the historical context and current challenges faced by the LGBTQ+ community. By providing compassionate and inclusive care, healthcare professionals can contribute to the overall health and well-being of homosexual individuals.

Legal protections for LGBTQ+ individuals

Legal protections for LGBTQ+ individuals have been a significant area of progress in recent years, providing crucial safeguards against discrimination and promoting equal rights and opportunities. In this subchapter, we will explore the legal landscape and progress made in terms of LGBTQ+ rights and protections, both globally and within specific countries.

One of the most significant advancements in LGBTQ+ rights is the legalization of same-sex marriage. Many countries, including the United States, have recognized the right of homosexual individuals to marry, granting them the same legal and financial benefits as opposite-sex couples. This landmark decision has brought immense joy and relief to countless LGBTQ+ individuals and couples, affirming their love and commitment.

However, despite these advancements, it is important to acknowledge that legal protections can vary significantly from one country to another.

In some nations, homosexuality is still criminalized, and LGBTQ+ individuals face persecution and discrimination. Healthcare workers must be aware of these disparities and advocate for the rights and well-being of LGBTQ+ individuals within their respective contexts.

In addition to marriage equality, many countries have implemented laws to protect LGBTQ+ individuals from discrimination in various areas of life, including employment, housing, education, and healthcare. These laws aim to ensure that homosexual individuals are treated fairly and have equal access to opportunities and services.

Furthermore, transgender rights have also gained significant attention in recent years. Many countries have enacted legislation to protect the rights of transgender individuals, including the right to legal recognition of gender identity, access to healthcare services, and protection against discrimination.

Despite these legal protections, challenges and barriers persist. LGBTQ+ individuals continue to face discrimination, violence, and stigma, both within society and within healthcare systems. Healthcare workers play a vital role in addressing these challenges by providing culturally competent and inclusive care to LGBTQ+ patients, advocating for policy changes, and ensuring that LGBTQ+ individuals are aware of their rights and legal protections.

In conclusion, legal protections for LGBTQ+ individuals have made significant progress in recent years, but there is still much work to be done. Healthcare workers have a crucial role in advocating for equal rights and providing inclusive care to LGBTQ+ individuals. By understanding the legal landscape and staying informed about the rights and protections available, healthcare workers can contribute to creating a more equitable and inclusive society for all.

Future trends and challenges in LGBTQ+ legislation

In recent years, there have been significant strides in LGBTQ+ rights and legislation, with many countries recognizing and protecting the rights of homosexual individuals. However, there are still several future trends and challenges that healthcare workers need to be aware of when it comes to LGBTQ+ legislation.

One of the key trends to watch out for is the continued push for comprehensive anti-discrimination laws. While progress has been made in many countries, there are still gaps in protection for LGBTQ+ individuals, particularly in areas such as employment, housing, and public accommodations. Healthcare workers need to advocate for the inclusion of sexual orientation and gender identity as protected categories in anti-discrimination laws to ensure equal access to healthcare and other essential services for LGBTQ+ individuals.

Another important trend is the increasing recognition of transgender rights. As transgender individuals continue to gain visibility and assert their rights, healthcare workers need to stay informed about the specific healthcare needs and challenges faced by this population. This includes issues related to gender-affirming healthcare, mental health support, and access to appropriate and respectful healthcare services.

Additionally, healthcare workers should be prepared for potential challenges related to religious exemptions and conscience clauses. While it is important to respect the diverse beliefs and values of healthcare providers, it is equally important to ensure that these exemptions do not lead to discrimination or the denial of care for LGBTQ+ individuals. Healthcare workers need to be knowledgeable about their legal obligations to provide respectful and inclusive care, regardless of their personal beliefs.

Furthermore, global trends and challenges in LGBTQ+ legislation should also be considered. While progress has been made in many countries, there are still places where homosexuality is criminalized, and

LGBTQ+ individuals face significant discrimination and violence. Healthcare workers can play a crucial role in advocating for the decriminalization of homosexuality and supporting initiatives to promote LGBTQ+ rights globally.

In conclusion, while there have been significant advancements in LGBTQ+ legislation, there are still future trends and challenges that healthcare workers need to be aware of. By staying informed, advocating for comprehensive anti-discrimination laws, recognizing transgender rights, navigating religious exemptions responsibly, and engaging in global LGBTQ+ advocacy, healthcare workers can contribute to creating a more inclusive and equitable healthcare system for all individuals, regardless of sexual orientation or gender identity.